Oncology

By

Dr. Steve J. Hayes

Table Of Contents

Oncology 1

Introduction 4

Chapter 1 5

Oncology 5

Chapter 2 11

Otolaryngology 11

Chapter 3 22

hematology oncology 22

Conclusion 29

Introduction

Oncology is the part of medication that includes the anticipation, conclusion, therapy, and investigation of malignant growth. Disease portrays the strange development of cells that outcomes in a huge mass known as a cancer.

Chapter 1

Oncology

The term oncology in a real sense implies a part of science that arrangements with growths and diseases. "Onco" means mass, mass, or disease while "- logy" connotes study.

What is infection?

Every one of the cells of the body has a firmly directed framework that controls their development, development, propagation, and possible demise. The disease starts when cells in a piece of the body begin to outgrow control. There are numerous sorts of diseases, yet they all start on account of the wild development of unusual cells.

How normal is malignant growth?

Today, a great many individuals are living with malignant growth or have had the disease. Malignant growth is the subsequent driving reason for death in the US. Around one-half of all men and 33% of all ladies in the US will foster malignant growth during their lifetimes.

How long has the disease existed?

The absolute earliest proof of malignant growth is found among fossilized bone cancers, human mummies in antiquated Egypt, and old compositions. Peculiarities suggestive of the bone dangerous development called osteosarcoma have been tracked down in mummies.

Among compositions, the main known portrayal of disease is found in the Edwin Smith Papyrus and is a duplicate of part of an old Egyptian reading material on injury medical procedure. It portrays 8 instances of growths or ulcers of the bosom that were treated by burning with a device called the fire drill. It traces back to around 3000 BC. . The papyrus portrays the condition as "serious".

The job of an oncologist

Clinical experts who practice oncology are called Disease trained professionals or oncologists. These oncologists play a few explicit parts. They help in the conclusion of the malignant growth, help in organizing the disease, and evaluate the forceful idea of the malignant growth.

Oncology analytic instruments

The main analytic instrument stays the clinical history of the patient. Normal side effects that point towards malignant growth incorporate weakness, weight reduction, unexplained sickliness, fever of obscure beginning, and so on.

Oncology relies upon analytic devices like biopsy or expulsion of pieces of cancer tissue and inspecting it under the magnifying lens. Other analytic devices incorporate endoscopy for the gastrointestinal parcel, imaging concentrates on X-beams, CT examining, X-ray checking, ultrasound, and other radiological procedures, Scintigraphy, Single Photon Outflow Figured

Tomography, Positron discharge tomography and atomic medication methods, and so on.

Normal techniques incorporate blood tests for natural or growth markers. Ascent of these markers in blood might be demonstrative of the disease.

Disease treatment

In light of the grade and phase of the malignant growth, oncologists assist with arranging the treatment that is appropriate for every one of their patients. This could be by a medical procedure, chemotherapy, radiation treatment, and different modalities.

Differently trained professionals

Therapy of disease might include different experts too. This incorporates a specialist, a radiation oncologist, or a radiotherapist and so forth the entire of the malignant growth treatment anyway is coordinated by the oncologists.

Backslide and abatement

When beginning treatment is finished the oncologist is answerable for follow-up of the patient to distinguish backslide and reduction. The previous means repeat or return of the disease while being abating implies remaining malignant growth free.

Palliative consideration

The oncologist is additionally liable for palliative or suggestive consideration in patients with terminal malignancies. This and different issues of treatment decisions have a few moral issues including patient independence and decision that the oncologist should be worried about.

Malignant growth screening

Oncology and malignant growth research include evaluating everybody for disease and screening the family members of patients (in sorts of malignant growth that are remembered to have a genetic premise. For instance, in bosom malignant growth both populace screening by normal mammography and familial screening by hereditary examination of the BRCA1 and BRCA2 qualities is performed.

Progress in oncology

A huge measure of exploration is being led in all areas of oncology, going from malignant growth cell science to chemotherapy treatment regimens and ideal palliative consideration and help with discomfort. This makes oncology a persistently changing and creating field.

Malignant growth research is completed in clinical preliminaries. In the UK, patients are much of the time signed up for huge examinations composed by Disease Exploration UK (CRUK), the Clinical Exploration Chamber (MRC), the European Association for Exploration and Therapy of Malignant Growth (EORTC), or the Public Disease Exploration Organization (NCRN).

Chapter 2

Otolaryngology

Otorhinolaryngology
(/oʊtoʊˌraɪnoʊˌlærɪnˈɡɒlədʒi/gracious toh-RY-noh-
LARR-in-GOL-ə-jee, condensed ORL and furthermore
known as otolaryngology, otolaryngology - head and neck
a medical procedure (ORL-H&N or OHNS), or ear, nose,
and throat (ENT) is a careful subspeciality inside
medication that arrangements with the careful and clinical
administration of states of the head and neck. Specialists
who represent considerable authority in this space are
called otorhinolaryngologists, otolaryngologists, head and
neck specialists, or ENT specialists or doctors. Patients
search for treatment from an otorhinolaryngologist for
sicknesses of the ear, nose, throat, base of the skull, head,
and neck. These normally incorporate practical infections
that influence the faculties and exercises of eating,
drinking, talking, breathing, gulping, and hearing.
Likewise, ENT medical procedure includes the careful

administration of diseases and harmless cancers and remaking of the head and neck along with plastic medical procedures of the face and neck.

Etymology

The term is a mix of Neo-Latin joining structures (oto-+ rhino-+ laryngo-+ - logy) got from four Old Greek words: οὖς ous (gen.: ὠτός otos), "ear", ῥίς rhis, "nose", λάρυγξ larynx, "larynx" and - λογία logia, "study" (cf. Greek ωτορινολαρυγγολόγος, "otorhinolaryngologist").

Training

Otorhinolaryngologists are doctors (MD, DO, MBBS, MBChB, and so on) who complete both clinical school and a normal of 5-7 years of post-graduate careful preparation in ORL-H&N. In the US, learners complete no less than five years of careful residency training. This contains three to a half years of general careful preparation and four and a half years in ORL-H&N expert medical procedure. In Canada and the US, experts complete a five-year residency preparing after clinical school.

Following residency preparation, some otolaryngologist-head and neck specialists complete a high-level sub-specialty partnership, where preparation can be one to two years in span. Partnerships incorporate head and neck careful oncology, facial plastic medical procedure, rhinology and sinus medical procedure, neuro-otology, pediatric otolaryngology, and laryngology. In the US and Canada, otorhinolaryngology is perhaps the most cutthroat specialty in medication where to get a residency position following clinical school

In the Unified Realm, access to higher careful preparation is serious and includes a thorough public choice process. The preparation program comprises 6 years of higher careful preparation after which students habitually embrace partnerships in a sub-specialty before turning into an expert.

The common absolute length of instruction, preparation, and post-auxiliary school is 12-14 years. Otolaryngology is among the more exceptionally remunerated careful claims to fame in the US. In 2023, the normal yearly pay was $118,230.

Themes by subspecialty

- Head and neck a medical procedure
- Head and neck careful oncology (field of a medical procedure treating disease/harm of the head and neck)
- Head and neck mucosal danger (malignant growth of the pink covering of the upper aerodigestive parcel)
- Oral disease (malignant growth of lips, gums, tongue, hard sense of taste, cheek, floor of mouth)
- Oropharyngeal disease (malignant growth of oropharynx, delicate sense of taste, tonsil, the base of tongue)
- Larynx disease (voice box malignant growth)
- Hypopharynx disease (lower throat malignant growth)
- Sinonasal disease
- Nasopharyngeal disease
- Skin disease of the head and neck

- Thyroid disease
- Salivary organ disease
- Head and neck sarcoma
- The endocrine medical procedure of the head and neck
- Thyroid medical procedure
- Parathyroid medical procedure
- Microvascular free-fold reconstructive medical procedure
- Skull base a medical procedure
-

Otology and neurotology

Fundamental articles: Otology and Neurotology

Investigation of illnesses of the external ear, center ear and mastoid, and inward ear, and encompassing designs, (for example, the facial nerve and horizontal skull base)

External ear sicknesses

- Otitis externa -
- outside ear or ear stream disturbance

- Focus ear and mastoid contaminations
- Otitis media - focus ear exacerbation
- Punctured eardrum (opening in the eardrum because of contamination, injury, blast, or boisterous commotion)
- Mastoiditis

Inward ear sicknesses

- BPPV - harmless paroxysmal positional dizziness
- Labyrinthitis/Vestibular neuronitis
- Ménière's sickness/Endolymphatic hydrops
- Perilymphatic fistula
- Acoustic neuroma, vestibular schwannoma

Facial nerve sickness

- Idiopathic facial paralysis (Ringer's Paralysis)

Facial nerve growths

- Ramsay Chase Disorder

Side effects

- Hearing misfortune
- Tinnitus (abstract commotion in the ear)
- Aural totality (feeling of completion in the ear)
- Otalgia (torment alluding to the ear)
- Otorrhea (liquid depleting from the ear)
- Dizziness
- Irregularity

Rhinology

Rhinology incorporates nasal brokenness and sinus illnesses.

- Nasal impediment
- Nasal septum deviation
- Sinusitis - intense, persistent
- Ecological sensitivities
- Rhinitis
- Pituitary growth
- Void nose disorder
- Serious or intermittent epistaxis

Pediatric otorhinolaryngology

- Adenoidectomy
- Acidic ingestion
- Cricotracheal resection
- Decannulation
- Laryngomalacia
- Laryngotracheal reproduction
- Myringotomy and cylinders
- Obstructive rest apnea - pediatric
- Tonsillectomy

Laryngology

Primary article: Laryngology

- Dysphonia/raspiness
- Laryngitis
- Reinke's edema
- Vocal string knobs and polyps
- Fitful dysphonia
- Tracheostomy
- Disease of the larynx
- Vocology - science and practice of voice habilitation

Facial plastic and reconstructive surgery

Facial plastic and reconstructive medical procedure is a one-year partnership open to otorhinolaryngologists who wish to start learning the tasteful and reconstructive careful standards of the head, face, and neck spearheaded by the specialty of Plastic and Reconstructive Medical procedure.

- Rhinoplasty and septoplasty
- Facelift (rhytidectomy)
- Browlift
- Blepharoplasty
- Otoplasty
- Genioplasty
- Injectable restorative medicines
- Injury to the face
- Nasal bone crack
- Mandible crack
- Orbital crack
- Front-facing sinus crack
- Complex slashes and delicate tissue harm
- Skin disease (for example Basal Cell Carcinoma)

Microvascular recreation repair

Microvascular recreation fix is a typical activity that is finished on patients who see an Otorhinolaryngologist. A microvascular reproduction fix is a surgery that includes moving a composite piece of tissue from the patient's body and moving it to the head as well as the neck. Microvascular head and neck recreation is utilized to treat head and neck malignant growths, including those of the larynx and pharynx, oral pit, salivary organs, jaws, calvarium, sinuses, tongue, and skin. The tissue that is generally normally moved during this technique is from the arms, legs, and back, and can emerge out of the skin, bone, fat, and additionally muscle. While doing this method, the choice on which is not entirely set in stone on the reconstructive necessities. Move of the tissue to the head and neck permits specialists to remake the patient's jaw, streamline tongue capability, and reproduce the throat. At the point when the bits of tissue are moved, they require their own blood supply for an opportunity of endurance in their new area. After the medical procedure is finished, the veins that feed the tissue relocate are reconnected to fresh blood vessels in the neck. These veins are ordinarily something like 1 to 3 millimeters in width which implies these associations should be made with a magnifying lens which is the reason this technique is designated "microvascular medical procedure.

Chapter 3

hematology oncology

What is hematology-oncology?

Hematology is the investigation of the physiology of blood and the sicknesses related to it and oncology is the investigation of a wide range of malignant growth.

Hematology-oncology is the cross-over of these two expert parts of medication worried about diagnosing, treating, and concentrating on diseases of the platelets, bone marrow, and related tissues. 'Blood diseases' incorporate leukemia (unreasonable unusual white cells in the blood), lymphoma, and myeloma (which can regularly incorporate an irregularity or growth comprised of strange white cells).

Various terms are utilized corresponding to disease, including 'neoplastic' change (and that implies strange new development) and 'threat' or dangerous, which alludes to something that is continuously and progressively seriously destructive - conceivably prompting difficult ailment or passing.

The term harmless is utilized to show something innocuous or just negligibly destructive. So the term 'harmless neoplasm' signifies a strange, yet moderately innocuous bump, while a 'threatening cancer' might be exceptionally hurtful in the event that it can develop and, spread through the body.

Hematologists and oncologists each go through expert preparation in the other field due to the cross-over and close relationship between the two clinical disciplines. 'Hematologist-oncologists' are the specialists from one or the other hematology or oncology who work in this field, treating patients and undertaking study and research to further develop care.

What is pediatric hematology-oncology?

Pediatric hematology-oncology is a further specialism of hematology-oncology zeroed in on diagnosing and treating kids with hematological diseases.

This is a significant clinical discipline, as youngsters and adolescents have exceptional clinical necessities. By and large, malignant growth is more normal with more seasoned age, yet a few especially testing tumors happen in youngsters, frequently connected with hematology. A portion of the distinctions in needs are physical as their bodies are as yet developing. Notwithstanding, a considerable lot of the clinical necessities of youngsters and teenagers are mental and close to home since they express their interests and considerations contrastingly to grown-ups.

Along these lines, pediatric hematologist-oncologists are prepared to be particularly understanding and skilled to ensure their young patients feel open to helping out with testing and treatment.

When to counsel a hematologist-oncologist?

There are different side effects that can be related to each sort of blood disease or turmoil. They can be explicit, like persevering irregularities in the neck or crotch north of a while (at the site of lymph hubs) or they can be very obscure or vague, like relentless sleepiness, migraines, or sickness. More often than not, normal and obscure side effects are not an indication of difficult sickness.

Notwithstanding, in the event that your Essential Consideration specialist alludes you to a hematology-oncology subject matter expert, this might be on the grounds that they wish to be wary and suspect the chance of a blood disease requiring expert examination. Being alluded to a hematologist-oncology doesn't guarantee to mean you have the disease and a significant part of the time this includes basically precluding the chance of danger via cautious assessment, blood testing, assessment of bone marrow, and imaging, like sweeps.

At the point when you visit a specialist who has some expertise in hematology-oncology, they will evaluate you and run a scope of tests to sort out the main driver of your side effects. These outcomes might turn out to be consoling, yet assuming the outcomes show that there is the chance of neoplastic change (destructive change) in the blood, delicate tissues, or bones, then the hematologist-oncologist will complete furthermore definite tests and start gathering a treatment plan.

What amount of time are blood tests required in an oncology office?

The time required to circle back for a blood test relies upon variables like the kind of test and the area of the test.

A total blood count (CBC), which estimates 19 boundaries of blood, is normally accessible to your PCP in 24 hours or less. The CBC is a generally utilized and significant blood test that can give significant hints or consolation about what might occur. It can show whether the different kinds of white cell counts are typical, strangely raised, or low, for instance.

A more unambiguous blood test giving more point-by-point data as a component of the check for malignant growth might take more time, especially in the event that you're getting a more uncommon blood test, for example, for specific immunoglobulins or cancer markers. These tests can require days to possibly more than seven days before results are accessible.

With the new approach of purpose in care CBC testing, sitting tight times for CBC can now be a lot more limited, with results regularly accessible within 10-12 minutes. These outcomes can be a fundamental sign that the blood framework is inside typical cutoff points or on the other hand that something is strange and requires clarification or further examination by your primary care physician.

How does a blood test assist with treating tumors?

A blood test is a significant part of diagnosing diseases. A total blood count assists the hematology-oncology expert with understanding on the off chance that any sorts of platelet are at an exhausted or raised level. For example, an unusually high white platelet count can demonstrate the chance of leukemia, which is a strangely unnecessary creation of specific sorts of white platelets.

The CBC and other standard tests, for example, liver capability tests, likewise give a sign of whether there is any proof of different impacts on the body, for example, iron deficiency or liver harm, that might have been brought about by a potentially malignant growth.

Following a total blood count, a specialist might arrange further, more unambiguous testing to limit the reason for the side effects and to check for specific prospects. These could incorporate blood protein testing to recognize unusual proteins brought about by malignant growth. Another successive investigation is a growth marker test, which can feature the chance of particular sorts of harmful cancer.

Frequently, the result of a starter round of tests can assist the specialist with realizing which further tests to arrange, to circle back to the underlying outcomes. Having the option to make a conclusion immediately can be useful in settling on a treatment plan. By and large, the sooner a conclusion can be made, the previous treatment can be begun, and the better the viewpoint for the patient.

Conclusion

An arrangement for the conclusion and therapy of malignant growth is a critical part of any general disease control plan. Its fundamental objective is to fix disease patients or draw out their life significantly, guaranteeing a decent personal satisfaction.